Psych Yourself Skinny

Sharon Geisen Hayes

(a gift from one FAT friend to another)

TO: _____

FROM: _____

Psych Yourself Skinny

Sharon Geisen Hayes

Hayes Productions LLC

Find us on the web at:

psychyourselfskinny.com
hayeslimited.com
hayesfinearts.com

PUBLISHED & PRINTED IN THE U.S.A.

Slightly Edited by Brandi Wills
Book Design & Illustrations by Sharon M Hayes

ISBN 978-0-615-16730-5

Psych Yourself Skinny Copyright © 2007 Sharon M Hayes All Rights Reserved. No part of this work may be reproduced or transmitted in any form whatsoever or by any means, electronic or mechanical, including photocopying and recording without written consent from artist/author Sharon M Hayes.

Other books in the works
by Sharon Geisen Hayes:

"Bobbie" *based on an actual account...*
When I interviewed my son's nanny (who I hired over the phone), she told me she was sane and had no bad habits or health problems, but she in fact had narcolepsy (can't stay awake), bone cancer, breast cancer, osteoporosis, was afraid of the dark, drank 22 cups of coffee a day, smoked like a chimney, cursed like a sailor, thought she was a psychic and is now dead. God love her, I miss her.

"Tar Bubbles" *an autobiography...*
"Bless me Father for I have sinned. My last confession was a few days before yesterday, which was the 4th of July 1966. These are my sins: I lied. I said some bad words. Last time I was here I forgot to confess that I accidentally stole a drumstick ice cream bar from old man Reins' grocery store because I didn't have enough money since I only stole one dime from my dad's change bag, which was only enough to pay for the sunflower seeds and the Zero candy bar. I cheated playing cards with my little brother Roy and took his money. I traded my First Holy Communion prayer book, rosary, Holy cards, pin, purse with the pretty white silk flowers on it and that doily thing for my head that Mom makes me wear in church, all for a plastic camera from rich Kathy in my class. Oh, and my fat cousin Johnny and I blew up all of the frogs in my grandma's pond yesterday with gunpowder we dug out of the leftover firecrackers we found. That's about it, I think."

IV

CONTENTS

Dedications.......page 1

Introduction.......page 3

The "Creative Bridge".......page 5

Learn to Laugh.......page 9

The Awful Truth.......page 11

Preparation.......page 17

Day Before Starting Day #1.......page 25
(psych session)

Your New "SKINNY ME" Routine.......page 31

Daily Meditations.......page 35

Everyday "SKINNY ME".......page 63
Meals in Minutes

"Don't be a Pig about it!".......page 71
Portion Control Chart

You Make the Choice.......73

VI

DEDICATIONS

I dedicate this book to two of the most beautiful soon-to-be skinny people in my life...

My loving mother Bernadine Geisen, who truly has reason to be overweight because she has had nine wild children, has had to diet most of her adult life and now fights diabetes and high cholesterol (my dad is skinny with high blood pressure and sneaks off to eat fried chicken gizzards and giant chocolate bars when mom is not looking). She is the epitome of a multitasking person and also had the quickest hand in the Midwest. She could drive an automobile and at the same time reach into the back seat and in one quick motion deservingly slap all five of us before we had time to duck. She also has the biggest and softest heart ever, and though there were nine of us, we never felt short changed in the love department. I love you Mom! And you too, Dad!

And secondly my big bad cousin Johnny Brinkman who used to blow up frogs with me down at our grandparents' pond when we were children (yes, we've gone to confession...well I know I have anyway.) Johnny is on a liquid diet, and it's not beer, so he can lose enough weight to have a hip replacement...Go Johnny! And read this entire book!!

2

INTRODUCTION

I'm standing at a check-out counter at the grocery store with yet another diet book in my hand. I give the book to the skinny, young checkout clerk. After quickly studying it she asks me if it was supposed to be a good diet. Not wanting her or any other clerk to think that I am fat because I am lazy or that I overindulge, I use my auto response: "Who knows, I just had a baby and I am going to try every diet I can get my fat hands on." She then surprises me with a question: "Oh, how old is your baby?" And without thinking it through I give her my honest answer: "Four years old." She laughs, and when I realize why she is laughing, I also realize that none of the other clerks had ever posed that question to me. She thought I was joking. I thought she was too damn nosey.

We are all born with the same amount of God given "self" power, but we are unique in how we train and use that power. I am a firm believer that you can achieve anything you want by putting your mind to it... Choose it, Claim it and Attain it. Life is what you make it...make it a bright one and most important, set your "self" goals for an even brighter future beyond this life, because your "self" is what carries on.

Turning FAT at age 40…

…My M.D. told me I could be a depressed bipolar or that it may be stress induced, but I have insisted on going untreated.

…My Endocrinologist told me that I am just going to be fat…it is in my genes.

… I asked my husband and truly my best friend if I was beginning to look like a side of beef. He replied, in the kindest way he knew how, "Well I wouldn't gain any more weight if I were you."

…My friends tell me muscle just weighs more than fat…let's go have a margarita and you'll feel better.

…My 13 year old son said, "Face it mom, you're FAT."

So, *if you want an honest opinion, go ask a kid, or an old person, because they know they can be honest and you won't punch their lights out.*

CHAPTER ONE

The "Creative Bridge"

Anybody can stick to a diet for at least a week or two, that's no problem. The problem is that if you don't see immediate results within the two weeks you get frustrated and quit, or you get bored with the type of diet you are on and quit. This book and routine is a 28-day deal. You cannot afford to quit it, because you will see results and you will have the proper tools to get you through the 28 days …just in time to do it another 28 days if you need it.

When I use the word "skinny," I don't mean bony thin. This word is used loosely here because when I was growing up, if a person was thin, we used the word "Skinny" and if a person was heavy we used the word "Fat." I guess as children we just took things down to their simplest forms. So I suppose the word skinny is a vocabulary habit for me and will be with me from now on, especially since we grew up with sayings like: "Skinny and Fatty were lying in bed, Fatty rolled over and Skinny was dead."

When my son was five years old, he and I were driving down our street and noticed my neighbor Bill walking alongside the road. He was noticeably thinner than he had been, so I pulled over, rolled down the window

5

and yelled "hey skinny, you're looking great." A couple of weeks later we were getting ready to leave for a Halloween party at another neighbor's house and my son asked me if "skinny" was going to be there… it took me a while to figure out what he was talking about. Then I realized that he thought Bill's name was Skinny. I just love how the mind works, especially when it is young and uncluttered.

So, do you want to be SKINNY or FAT? Make a choice and stick with it. Right now.

When I decided on my career as a creative director, it was because I wanted to do something that I enjoyed. It has been a success because of the enjoyment.

To be successful at something, you need a "creative bridge" between what you want to do and what you do. If you do something you enjoy, you will stay focused and give it your full attention. This same formula applies to everything you do…If you don't like something about yourself and you want to make a successful change, you will need to "create" an enjoyable way to make that change.

Here is a sample of my process for building a "creative bridge" which has turned out to be the premise for creating this book…

What do I want to change about myself? Answer: I want to be back to my skinny self.

I already know that weight gain is caused by two main factors: Eating more calories than your body can burn off and/or not eating the right types of foods.

Well, I usually make healthy food choices when I eat, with the exception of that one girly time of the month when the aliens land, possess my body and I lose all mental reasoning between good and bad everything. But unless I am on a photo or video shoot, my job consists of sitting in brainstorming meetings, behind a computer or standing behind an art easel for very long hours at a time.

So the problem is that I do not burn off more calories than I take in, which means I will need to exercise to burn off excess calories.

I'm not really big on hitting the exercise mat. I sometimes get bored with working out in a gym, and I totally suck at aerobics.

What do I like to do in the form of exercise? Answer: I like to freestyle dance. I also enjoy tennis but that requires a partner. So to help my body burn off the extra calories I will need to dance. My **"creative bridge"** between fat and skinny is **"dance."**

Freestyle dance is fun. It is also a stress reliever. Dance is something you can do anytime anywhere and it does not cost money. You don't even have to get dressed for it.

The more you move your body the more you burn. On day one of this book I will give you some great freestyle dance tips, which will optimize the toning of your body. If you don't like to dance, just move around.

Your **"creative bridge"** may be brisk walking, riding a bike or being creative with the types of meals you incorporate into your daily menu.

CHAPTER TWO

Learn to Laugh

Michael Ankelman, a great writer friend of mine, is always giving me his versions of famous sayings, and this one has always made me laugh:

"When you laugh the world laughs with you. When you cry the world laughs at you."

One of the key tools in this book is to laugh with each other and at each other, and never cry unless it stems from too much laughter. This life is too short to be sad about how much we weigh, yet it is long enough for us to make a positive change about the way we eat, how we exercise and our attitude towards it. Be Happy.

Unlike the skinny authors of other diet books who have "before" and "after" shots shown in their books, because they were inspired to write after their diet journey, I don't have an "after" picture. I am a 47 year old FAT Creative Director on a mission to get skinny, which won't happen until I get this book written and have a chance to read and follow it.

Today I saw an old friend who has not seen me since I've become fat…so I used this book as an excuse and told him that I had to gain 50 pounds so I could write this book. When I end up on some TV talk show I will be thin, I promise, and it will be because of this crazy, in-your-face and on-your-mind book.

This book is not going to talk to you about all of the medical reasons why you should lose weight, because if that type of psychology really worked we'd already be thin.

I'm also not going to give you one of those charts that tell you how much you should weigh. We both know we need to lose weight...dwelling on how much can be overwhelming and depressing...we want to look at the lighter side of being fat and lose it with laughter in a new and creative way.

This book will stimulate your thought process with thought-provoking mental visuals related to your FAT self. You may laugh yourself skinny or be so disgusted that you can't eat. There will also be daily writing lessons included in this program. For this to work properly you MUST NOT SKIP a lesson! And finally a very blunt meditation for each day to help you psych yourself skinny with me.

Take a moment now to view what I like to refer to as my "Don't be a Pig about it" Portion Control Chart and the "No need to Sneak It!" Snack Guide found in the back of this book. You may want to cut these out and hang them on your fridge. This is about as technical as it gets in this book.

CHAPTER THREE

The Awful Truth

In 1988 I owned and drove a **Porsche**. I weighed 123 lbs. Today I drive a **big fat van** and I am 50 lbs. heavier. I think there may be a subliminally forced "filling of the space" going on here.

Could you hold a garage sale just for your diet book collection? I could, and I did.

Did you stop buying new clothes when you realized you went up another size and refused to give into your body? Instead, you started buying more accessories... And the bigger they were the smaller you felt? Too bad big hair is out of style, it did make the butt look smaller. I was in denial about having a weight problem for a long time, because I could hide it pretty well under big floppy scarves, or so I thought.

I'll never forget the first time I realized I must look fat to other people. I was standing at a jewelry counter, in a very bad mood, buying yet another BIG piece of jewelry when out of the corner of my eye, I quickly caught the side view of this expressionless FAT lady down at the end of the counter staring at me. I thought to myself, what are you lookin' at fatty? When I turned to leave I realized that what I thought was another

11

person was one of those poles with a mirror slapped on it...What a brutal awakening! I started laughing at myself for calling myself a fatty, then I cried all the way to my car.

Does it take you an hour or two to find something that looks just "ok" to put on before heading out to an event with friends, or you cancel going altogether because you are not your skinny self and are so depressed and embarrassed about the way you look? I end up mummified. Once I skipped a really close friend's funeral all because I didn't want the people who had not seen me in years to see me as my fat self. I really regret that I didn't go, and that I let my fat self get the best of me...to top it off the friend who died probably never weighed under 300 pounds his entire adult life, which never bothered me, I love fat people.

Are the majority of the clothes in your closet either hangy black or the old skinny ones? You're thinking, I will get back into this. You're probably also thinking that you're going to have a chance to burn the fat ones before you die and hide the evidence...just like those pictures you cut yourself out of or pitched before anyone else got to see them. I think this is a girl thing...do guys do this? Have you ever seen a man cut his picture out because he thought he looked too fat?

Do you start a diet full of enthusiasm the first day and start cheating within the first week or two, only to find yourself saying, "Well maybe this one is not for me. I'll try another one tomorrow or next week."

I am so good at creative cheating...I started one diet where you are suppose to lose weight if you stay within a certain amount of points. At the end of the day if I had eaten too many points...I would go back and erase some of my portion sizes in my little book thinking that if the points weren't written on that little paper they didn't count. Been there yet?

Then I tried the buddy workout system with my fat next door neighbor friend. Since I had all the equipment at my house we decided to get skinny there. Well you know how they say if you have a workout buddy you will keep each other motivated... We'd motivate each other to work out for 20 minutes every morning and then motivate each other to hit the fast food joint for a supreme croissant and a soda. Then, I'd have to drive her back to her house, next door, because she was too tired to walk it. That buddy thing works in two directions...my suggestion is that if you are going to have a workout buddy, make it a skinny, overachiever.

Then there were the hypnosis tapes...Ha! I won't even go there. I still use them when I'm having a hard time falling asleep.

When I tried a box of diet patches from the health food store, I didn't know that you are not suppose to change the patch each time you shower. I ended up with high blood pressure the following week, which only lasted for a few days once I figured out what I had done wrong. About the only thing I didn't try was surgery or drugs. I hate both, or else I probably would have.

The funniest weight loss gimmick I ever saw was when I was 19. A very thin friend of mine who always thought her thighs and butt were too big, bought this contraption that looked like a piece of silver plastic wrap with holes all over it. You'd wrap it around your fat body part, hook it up to the vacuum hose and flip the switch. I wish I would have taken a photo. This must have been the really early, really less invasive version of liposuction.

I never really had a weight problem before I turned 38. I always worked out and played tennis or racquetball.

When I was pregnant with my son, I hired a personal weight trainer, thinking that if I kept working out I would not have any problems getting back into shape once I gave birth. In my seventh month I told the trainer to hit the road and my dog Watson and I discovered the fast food taco stand down the road. I'd order a burrito supreme for myself and toss a floured tortilla into the back passenger seat for Watson. We ate one almost every day for the rest of my pregnancy. I gained about 36 pounds during my pregnancy. Within four months of giving birth I was back to my normal size again, mostly living on soup, playing tennis every day and doing a couple of six-day spring water only fasts. I felt great.

Then at age 39, I started picking up weight and not being able to get it back off. After the gain of 16 new pounds I tried another spring water fast, followed by a trip to an endocrinologist (a doctor who specializes in analyzing blood to see if there is any hidden problems going on).

The office nurse drew my blood and the tiny Chinese doctor told me everything looked great and that I need not worry. She said to pick up my exercise routine a bit and I should be fine, that my metabolism had probably just slowed down some.

OK, I purchased some new weight equipment and added three miles a day to my treadmill routine. That year I gained another 15 pounds. Then at age 40, I was 31 pounds over my normal weight. Off to see the wizard once more…more blood was drawn and then enters the Asian doctor skimming over my chart and glancing at me every so often. "So wet me see Sharwin…you come to see me last year and you thin, you look good, you thirty nine…Now you come to see me, you fat, unhappy, you forty, you look bad…Oh you forty, you just gonna be fat! Is in your genes. You gonna cry a lot, then you get angry a lot, then when you turn fifty-five or so you gonna go back to normal. Don't worry, you healthy."

Well I've got news for you Doc…I'm not waiting until I turn fifty-five to get skinny again.

Here we go…

16

CHAPTER FOUR

Preparation

We've all read enough good diet books to know what's healthy and what's not, but in case you've conveniently forgotten, here are a few tips on what to buy and what to remember as you prepare your meals throughout the day.

- **FOR A HEALTHY DAY EVERY DAY YOU SHOULD HAVE:** PROTEIN, CALCIUM, FRESH FRUITS & VEGETABLES, WHOLE GRAINS, SIX TO EIGHT CUPS OF WATER…. AND TAKE A MULTI-VITAMIN.

- Everything in moderation <u>IS NOT OK</u> if you don't know how to stick to the moderation part.

- Fresh is best! Next comes frozen, try to avoid canned foods or at least the ones with lots of sodium unless you're stocking a bomb shelter.

- Shop on the outside aisles of the grocery stores (this is where you will find the good, fresh, healthy foods).

- Try to avoid products made with white flour. Stick with whole grain or sprouted grain and gluten free products.

- Stay away from fake sugars and sweeteners…just use less of the real thing or a little honey.

- Use real butter, olive oils and canola oils in moderation.

- Green is great…try to get lots of green veggies.

- Fruit is a natural cleanser. Don't eat too much though, berries & grapefruits are best.

- Don't eat after 7p.m., or at least 3 hours before going to bed.

- Lemon or lime juice makes a great low-cal salad dressing

- Experiment with herbs and spices in your meal creations. Spicy foods can help curb the appetite.

- Use baked garlic, light soft cheese or cream cheese as a spread on your bread or toast instead of butter.

- If you enjoy drinking alcoholic beverages, limit yourself to one to three drinks per week…remember, alcohol slows down the metabolism and causes you to feel hungry when you are not, and it robs your body of good nutrients. Not to mention it is a waste of bad calories, which could be substituted for a healthy food item.

- Organic is the best choice for getting the most nutrients from fruits and vegetables.

- Don't overcook your vegetables, this will cook the nutrients out...try to steam them until they are bright in color.

- When you are buying eggs, get the ones with omega 3.

- Ground flaxseed or flaxseed oil is a great source of omega 3. Add a tablespoon to your smoothie or protein shake.

- Eat off of a smaller sized plate than you are used to.

- Don't eat if your not hungry.

- If dining out ask your waiter to have your food prepared to the "lighter" side. Avoid the breads or at least limit your bread intake to one slice and try to make it a whole grain slice. Also avoid other starches, unless it is whole grain, then just have a smaller amount than normal.

SKINNY ME PANTRY AND FRIDGE...Out with the fat me, in with the skinny me.

Throw away or give away all the "dead" food in your pantry and fridge...any chemically modified,

refined, fake fried, sugar loaded and coated junk that's hanging around…pitch it now. Right now…. Get up off your fat ass and do it NOW!

Below is a grocery list of items that make for good choices in everyday meal planning. If you have trouble finding them at your regular grocery store, ask the store manager to stock it…they will usually do this, otherwise your local health food store should have it:

- Whole Grain Melba Rounds

- Whole Sprouted Grain Breads or whole grain, low carb bread with omega 3 and flaxseed

- Whole Grain Tortillas

- Whole Grain English Muffins **TIP: Keep all of the bread items in the freezer and use as needed.**

- Cream of Wheat or Oatmeal (instant single-serve packs)

- "Gluten Free" Whole Grain pasta, beans, lentils, rice

- Eggs with Omega 3 **TIP: Always have some boiled eggs on hand for added protein to salads or for a healthy quick lunch or snack.**

- Real Peanut Butter, no added sugar

- Olive Oil, Canola Oil, Real Butter

- Fish …the less sodium or fat the better

- Meat cuts with the least amounts of fat: chicken, pork tenderloin, beef tenderloin, turkey

- Raw Nuts (limit yourself to 5-6 whole nuts per day)

- Fresh and Frozen Fruit

- Fresh and Frozen Vegetables

- Broccoli sprouts

- Skim Milk, Yogurt & Frozen Yogurt

- White Cheese, Cream Cheese, Light spreadable cheese

- Honey

- 100% all natural fruit spread sweetened only with fruit and fruit juice

- **Snack foods:** Popcorn or Baked Snack Food in single-serve sizes **TIP: (if you cannot find it in a single serve size, buy the regular size bag and then separate it into one cup servings in zipper baggies). There are several great tasting snack food alternatives in the health food department of the grocery stores, or at the health food stores. Check them out.**

- Chicken Broth and/or Beef Broth (LOW SODIUM)

- Spices, Herbs & Seasonings: fresh garlic, salt, pepper, cayenne pepper, basil, Montreal steak seasoning

- Sparkling Mineral Water…this comes in various flavors **TIP: try to avoid the ones with sugar in them. You are safest with lemon or lime flavors or you can add your own fresh lemon or lime. Force yourself to get use to drinking this if you normally drink soda. If you need a bit of something sweet in it at first, try a tablespoon of honey or a teaspoon of sugar.**

- Antioxidant loaded Tea. whatever flavor you prefer

- Lemons & Limes

Other Items:

- One spiral notebook and label it "Skinny Me" I've included 28 days of lined pages in the back of this book to get you started.

- Calendar
- Radio or CD player (if you want to dance or move it to the music)

Projecting your goal weight. Weigh yourself and record that weight on the Monday square of your calendar (your starting date in the calendar). On every Monday after that subtract three pounds from the weight of the Monday before and write it on every Monday until you get to your goal weight. This may require more than one calendar year, and you may end up losing more than three pounds a week…you can adjust your calendar as you drop the weight.

You can weigh yourself once a week to track your progress, but not more than once a week.

If I want to lose three to five pounds per week, I keep my calorie intake between 1,000 - 1,200 calories per day. Buy a calorie count guide if you want to keep track of your calories. Figure out how many calories you need per day for a healthy diet that will still allow you to lose those unwanted pounds. Here is a sample of how I split my calories up throughout the day:

> Breakfast – 300 cal
> 10 a.m. Snack – 75 cal
> Lunch – 350 cal
> 2 p.m. Snack – 75 cal
> Dinner – 300 cal
> 7 p.m. Snack – 100 cal

Here is an easy method for estimating your caloric needs (for healthy, non-pregnant adults age 18-50). Adults over the age of 50 should further reduce calories by 10% to 20%.

1. Set your realistic "Skinny Me" weight:_____.

2. Classify yourself by lifestyle.
LESS ACTIVE (little to no regular exercise, couch potato, lazy, or maybe a desk job) __13__.

ACTIVE (moderate level of regular exercise, 15-20 minute walk per day, active at work) __15__.

VERY ACTIVE (eye-bulging strenuous regular exercise, running, manual labor at work) __17__.

3. Multiply your "Skinny Me" weight by your activity level: _____ x _____ = _____ (this is the amount of daily calories needed to maintain your "Skinny Me" weight once you have reached it.)

4. Subtract 500 calories a day to lose one pound per week. Subtract 1,000 calories a day to lose two pounds per week, not to fall below 1,200 calories per day. 1,200 calories is the least amount of calories you can consume in one day before you run the risk of malnutrition. ___ (calories from step 3)___ - ___(500-1,000 calories to lose weight)___ = __(daily caloric goal)_____.

What's your goal weight?_____
What's your goal date?_____

24

CHAPTER FIVE

Day Before Starting Day #1

Psych Session: We all have a "skinny me" within us. She/he may not have seen the light of day for awhile but I can guarantee the skinny me is there. Imagine yourself as two persons, the skinny self on the inside and the fat self on the outside.

Today, stand in front of a full-length mirror naked and have a good laugh out loud as your fat self. Picture in your mind all of the things you did and how much fun you had creating your fat self. Think of all the soda, the beer or wine, the food & dessert feast with your friends, the extra taco, potato chip or pizza etc, etc.

Wiggle around and watch that blubber jiggle, pinch or grab a handful of that fat, and notice that there really is a bone structure underneath. Picture yourself in one-half-inch layers from the bone structure out. Within that first half-inch layer next to your hipbone is your skinny me.

While you are still standing there, close your eyes, be your skinny self now, and allow your skinny self inside to get focused. Dwell on all of those times when you were tormented, depressed, angry and cried because of that fat self. You now realize that your skinny self

25

needs to take control of the situation. Allow your skinny self to get angry at your fat self.

Open your eyes and look deep into your eyes until you see the determination of the "skinny me" within. Let your skinny self have a chat with your fat self...Say aloud, addressing your fat self in an angry tone:

"Look what you've done to me you selfish, foolish slob! You've been out there enjoying yourself while I'm trapped up in here taking all the heat and humiliation, not to mention doing all the worrying about my health and well being."

Now shake out that anger and say:

"That's it, I'm through with you, I'm in control now. You're out of here, I am coming out, and that is a promise!"

Just like a young child has to be taught and disciplined, so too does your fat self need to be taught and disciplined.

NOTE: If you are a fast food lover or a junk food junkie, you will want to do the following exercises before starting **Day One**.

The Power to Will or Won't. I like to think of this as strength training the mind, letting it know who is in charge. At breakfast or lunch when you are good and hungry, drive through your favorite fast food restaurant and let your fat self order what you want, along with a large glass of water, tea or coffee. If you only ordered a salad with your drink, then go ahead and eat and ignore what I am about to tell you. Chances are you bought a "bag-o-crap."

Pull your car into a vacant parking spot on that same lot. While sipping on your drink open the food container and examine that food very closely. Take a good whiff of it too…While doing this, think about all of the hidden and wasted calories, nasty artery-clogging fat and bad carbs that are in this tempting meal you just bought and the negative effects it will have on your BIG, FAT, Nutritionally Starved body. Close your eyes for a moment, picturing your skinny self inside and remember the promise "skinny me" made to yourself in the mirror. Now, take a big breath in through your nose and blow it back out your mouth, visualizing your skinny self and how you're going to dress once you climb out of that selfish fat self. You're in control… Remember your skinny self is in there, we just have to psych it back out! It is mind over matter…**remind yourself that no food tastes as good as you're going to look and feel in those skinny clothes.**

Now wrap **ALL** of that nasty food back up, get out of your car and take it to the nearest trash can. Before throwing it away, shake that bag in the air and as loud

27

as you can, yell out:

"I'm too good for this crap! I'm in control now."

Then drive back through and order something nutritional. The employees at the food establishment may think someone in the kitchen screwed up your order and to appease you give you the next order for free. If you're too embarrassed, just throw on a pair of sunglasses and disguise your voice.

THIS MAY SEEM A BIT DRASTIC, BUT REMEMBER...DESPERATION CALLS FOR DRASTIC MEASURES!

If you absolutely must eat your really bad choices, try ordering one good thing and one bad thing, then only eat a small amount of the bad thing. For example, order a small non-diet soda and a large iced tea or water. Sip just enough of the soda to get your fix then throw it away and drink the ice tea or water.

You could also try giving yourself an incentive. Put a jar on your desk at work, in your kitchen on top the refrigerator, or even in your car near the dash. Each time you want to hit the fast food track, hit a grocery store instead and have a deli sandwich of white meat on whole grain, an apple and a bottle of ice cold water or tea. Put the change in your jar. After one week treat yourself to a manicure, pedicure, facial, a pack of new golf balls, etc. You will be surprised at how much money you save when you substitute nutritional food for fast food.

If you dip into the chips a bit too much you may have to gross yourself out by taking a handful and putting them in a clear plastic bag. Next smash it up and then check out that nasty grease on the sides of the bag. Just think, that could be in your system clogging up your arteries or causing major damage to your beautiful complexion. Also, set a potato chip in a fire proof dish in the sink and light the chip with a match and watch how fast it burns up…poof! Just another testament to how much grease is involved here.

You might also try letting the chips sit out in a bowl for three days and then eat a big hand full of them, next time you return to the chip cabinet you'll have a different taste association with the product you're staring at.

For the sweet tooth, you could also trick that product-taste association response by putting some nasty tasting spice on that cake, or just take a lick of a deodorant stick and that will keep you from tasting anything. In fact, my next product creation may be a spray taste bud killer.

If you crave chocolate try this: Take a small bite of an unlit birthday candlestick, chew it and spit it out. Now take a bite of plain chocolate bar…notice a familiar taste? It's called paraffin (wax). Yuck…that is what helps chocolate hold its shape.

Soda Lover? Switch to sparkling mineral water, and to wean off of the sweet taste add a little honey, fresh

29

lemon or lime, or buy the all-natural fruit flavored variety with no added sugars or sugar substitutes. If you need a negative association to rid you of that soda habit, and the sugar content alone does not scare you, think of the acid and how it plays on your stomach. One of the things you're not supposed to drink if you have an ulcer or a hole in your stomach is soda... hmm...why do you think that is? Try storing your soda next to your household cleaning products for a couple of weeks, and each time you start to reach for a soda, grab a cleanser bottle and read it instead. Then go to the fridge or faucet and get yourself a nice glass of cold clear refreshing water...remember water is the best thing going when it comes to a drink...it's good for your skin and your health.

CHAPTER SIX

Your New "SKINNY ME" Routine

Tonight set your alarm clock to wake you up 30 minutes earlier than your normal wake up time.

What to look forward to EVERYDAY:

Daily Meditation
Before getting out of bed read your Daily Meditation. To get the most of your meditation you should recall it over and over throughout the day…it may help to write it out on a piece of paper and put it in your pocket or purse.

Everyday Morning Stretch and Wake-up Routine
UPON AWAKENING Take a big, long deep breath in through your nose and blow it back out of your mouth…do this three times slowly.

First thing out of bed do a morning stretch…
(A) Reach for the sky as high as you can, rocking up and down on your tiptoes. Back down flat on your feet with both arms still up in the air above your head, (B) stretch and reach one arm at a time like you are picking stars out of the sky directly above your head and pulling them down towards you. (C) Bring one

arm down and put that hand on your hip. Then do a side bend by bending at the waist and reaching over towards the side with the hand on the hip. Repeat this on the other side. (D) Now bend over to touch your toes or the closest thing you can reach to the toes, or until you feel a stretch up your backside. (E) Next, put one foot up on something solid like the side of your bathtub or a step and do a few knee bends on each leg. (F) Hold onto the back of a chair or the wall and stretch the thighs one at a time by bending your leg up behind you and grabbing onto your ankle or toe…pull your foot close to your buttocks and hold it there for 10 seconds, repeat with the other leg. Hold each of these positions for 10 seconds and repeat them three times.

Go to the mirror and look into the eyes of that "skinny me" and say: "Good morning." Then think about that promise and say: "Let's show them what we are made of. My skinny me is in control now, and I am coming out!"

Drink a big glass of water. Each time you are drinking a glass of water you should close your eyes while visualizing the cleansing process and how that water is carrying all of the impurities and toxins out of your system. Think to yourself… "in with the good, out with the bad."

Now turn on that music and start dancing...

Close your eyes and visualize your skinny self within. Also visualize that thin outfit you will be dressing in when you bring out your skinny self. Try to dance for at least 15 minutes. NOTE: You may want to move the furniture out of your way so your "Fat Self" does not break it.

NOTE: If you hate to dance just step in place to the music while waving your arms in a circular motion.

Freestyle Dance Tips
Getting started and optimizing the toning of your muscles being used while you dance.

• Once you decide on a room or area to be used for dancing, you can set the mood with dim lighting or candles.

• Any type of radio will work, however the best type will be a small boom box type. This will be easy to move from room to room or pack along on a trip if you need to. Headphones will limit your dance moves and keep you from moving about freely. If you must use headphones, use the small wireless kind or the type with the radio built into the earpiece.

• Be sure to keep a clock nearby so you will know how many minutes you have been dancing or moving.

• If you're feeling alone, dance in front of a mirror or invite another friend to dance with you.

• Dance barefoot if you are on a non-carpeted floor

or in your socks if you are on a carpeted floor, so you will have more control over your movements.

- Start off at a slower pace for the first three minutes so your body has a chance to warm up. Then let her rip!

- If the radio station takes a commercial break, keep dancing, don't stop.

- While you are swinging those arms, try pushing your reach just a little further than you normally would so that you can feel the stretch.

- Lift or kick your legs out in front of you during some of those dance moves.

- Bend at the knees and twist down into a squat, try to hold that position for a few seconds and then twist back to the upright position. NOTE: It does not have to be a deep squat...just go down far enough to fill the stretch in your thighs.

- Try holding in your stomach muscles when at all possible during your dance moves.

- Remember, the best tip of all is...The more you tune in and move it, the more you tone up!

Every night just before going to bed you will have a written lesson to put in your "skinny me" notebook.

34

CHAPTER SEVEN

Daily Motivational Meditations

DAY ONE (Monday)

Meditation for the day… If you think just because they're your friends they're not talking about how fat you are, your wrong. Even your fat friends are talking about how fat you are. Let's get up off our FAT butts and show them what we are made of, make this change with me today, so we can psych the fat off and bring out our skinny self! Before you know it they'll be gawking instead of talking.

WHAT'S YOUR GOAL WEIGHT? _____
WHAT'S YOUR GOAL DATE? _____

Skinny me notebook lesson
Before going to bed take out your "Skinny Me" diary and write:

I'm getting into shape. I'm in control. 20 times.

DAY TWO (Tuesday)

Meditation for the day…Remember you have a choice each time you put something into your mouth…make it a good choice. If you want to look like a doughnut or any other fat food, just keep eating them and you will. Or listen to your "skinny me," take that nutritional plunge and we'll get trim and healthy together.

WHAT'S YOUR GOAL WEIGHT? _____
WHAT'S YOUR GOAL DATE? _____

Skinny me notebook lesson
I DO NOT eat junk food. I'm in control.   20 times.

DAY THREE (Wednesday)

Meditation for the day…Your body is ALIVE…feed it natural LIVE FOOD…FRESH and healthy foods… not DEAD, chemically filled, processed food. Your complexion, hair, nails, skin…are a reflection of what goes into and onto your body. Keep it all alive and healthy looking.

WHAT'S YOUR GOAL WEIGHT? _____
WHAT'S YOUR GOAL DATE? _____

Skinny me notebook lesson
My skinny me is alive and in control.   20 times.

DAY FOUR (Thursday)

Meditation for the day…Your "Fat self" is always out to trip you up. Always have your "skinny me" one step ahead by having the good nutritional foods and snacks within reach for those hungry or weak moments.

WHAT'S YOUR GOAL WEIGHT? _____
WHAT'S YOUR GOAL DATE? _____

Skinny me notebook lesson
Skinny me is always a step ahead.   20 times.

DAY FIVE (Friday)

Meditation for the day…Some people may like cottage cheese, but no one likes cottage cheese legs. You need to stay focused on melting that fat off, layer by disgusting layer, and the only way to do that is to keep your Fat trap shut. Remember your skinny me is in control at all times.

WHAT'S YOUR GOAL WEIGHT? _____

WHAT'S YOUR GOAL DATE? _____

Skinny me notebook lesson
Shut up fatty, I'm in control.   20 times.

DAY SIX (Saturday)

Meditation for the day…Take your fat self outside today, to a park or the mall. Get a good look at all the fat people out there. Try to visualize what they would wear, how they would walk and what their facial expressions might be if they were skinny. Pretend they are all getting this same advice and that they are looking at you too. Go ahead, get out there. Chances are if you are still wearing your fat self on the outside you will laugh when you have eye contact with another fat person, and that's OK. Remember, that is your skinny self doing the laughing and we are laughing the fat self away.

WHAT'S YOUR GOAL WEIGHT? _____
WHAT'S YOUR GOAL DATE? _____

Skinny me notebook lesson
Laughter is healthy; being fat is not healthy.   20 times.

DAY SEVEN (Sunday)

Meditation for the day…Ah another great day for a dance. Today let's focus on God and all that God given control within our skinny self. Do you think God put you here to sit, eat, and get fat? I think not, so let's try refocusing our thoughts today on why God put us here. Sit down and write up your mission statement for your life, in other words why you think you are here on this earth. I don't see the word "Fat" in there, do you?

WHAT'S YOUR GOAL WEIGHT? _____

WHAT'S YOUR GOAL DATE? _____

Skinny me notebook lesson
My Skinny mission is to get out of the fat and into my skinny clothes. 20 times.

Before starting day EIGHT refer back to your psyche session and repeat the session again. You will do this at the beginning of every week.

DAY EIGHT (Monday)

Meditation for the day…Remember the bigger the car the smaller you look, however that's only when your sitting in it. The bigger the clothes the fatter you look, no matter how small you feel. Today try on a pair of your skinny pants and see how far up you get them. Hang them in an area of your home where you are forced to look at them several times a day. Every other day try to put them on, as though it were the only thing you have to wear. Look in the mirror and tell your fat self "I'll fit into these in a couple of days." It may seem redundant, however you will fit into them eventually if you listen to your "skinny me" and stay in control. Remember your skinny me has to retrain your mind and discipline your fat self, as though it were a child.

WHAT'S YOUR GOAL WEIGHT? _____
WHAT'S YOUR GOAL DATE? _____

Skinny me notebook lesson
Skinny me is in control. I am losing weight. 20 times.

42

DAY NINE (Tuesday)

Meditation for the day…If it feels wrong, it's wrong. Don't give in to your fat self and its nasty cravings. Be psyched and ready to say NO. Remember the promise your skinny me made to your fat self. If you're having trouble, grab a mirror and put it on your refrigerator.

WHAT'S YOUR GOAL WEIGHT? _____
WHAT'S YOUR GOAL DATE? _____

Skinny me notebook lesson
I'm coming out and that's a promise! 20 times.

DAY TEN (Wednesday)

Meditation for the day… Always feel self-conscious. Especially when you are eating in a restaurant. Even if nobody is looking at you, pretend they are. And if you are with your friends remember that they do talk behind your back about the things you put into your mouth. This will keep your fat self in check at all times. And remember, even when your fat self thinks no one is around, your skinny me is always there watching and ready to take control.

WHAT'S YOUR GOAL WEIGHT? _____
WHAT'S YOUR GOAL DATE? _____

Skinny me notebook lesson
I'm watching you fatty!   20 times.

DAY ELEVEN (Thursday)

Meditation for the day...Breathe. Close your eyes and breathe in all of that skinny air. Think about the time when there was no fat self. How light you felt, how you could breathe in your skinny clothes without feeling like you were being strangled at the waistline, neck or armholes. The best you felt. Today put on something that is tight and uncomfortable at the waist, neck and arms. Try to keep it on for at least one hour. Notice that awful choking feeling? This is to remind the fat self that there is still work to be done and that the skinny me is determined for these clothes to fit loose again.

WHAT'S YOUR GOAL WEIGHT? _____
WHAT'S YOUR GOAL DATE? _____

Skinny me notebook lesson
My clothes will not strangle me! 20 times.

DAY TWELVE (Friday)

Meditation for the day With your "skinny me" in control you will no longer have to fear, or have the embarrassments of tight spaces. When you are in your fat self think about all of the feelings evoked by the sight of a theater seat, ballgame seat, airline seat, café booth, theme park ride seat, a seat or chair with arms and an allocated area for your butt to fit in. Keep your skinny me in control and soon you'll be sitting comfortably anywhere.

WHAT'S YOUR GOAL WEIGHT? _____
WHAT'S YOUR GOAL DATE? _____

Skinny me notebook lesson
Skinny me is in control. I can sit anywhere. 20 times.

DAY THIRTEEN (Saturday)

Meditation for the day…Going out to an event or just hooking up with friends for dinner is so much more enjoyable without the stress of agonizing over what to wear because most of your dress clothes don't fit, look or feel right. When was the last time you wore your favorite dress or sports coat? Your "skinny me" is going to get you back into those great clothes. Take a look at your favorite clothes today, and take a trip to the mall and start selecting the types of clothes you will be wearing soon. If you are going out with friends tonight, keep your skinny me in control and during the course of the evening think about the things you will be wearing next time you meet up with this same group. If you're not going out tonight grab a stack of clothing catalogues or magazines and start clipping out the clothes you want to wear.

WHAT'S YOUR GOAL WEIGHT? _____
WHAT'S YOUR GOAL DATE? _____

Skinny me notebook lesson
Skinny me is in control and I look amazing. 20 times.

DAY FOURTEEN (Sunday)

Meditation for the day…Get out and be seen today because your skinny me is coming out! You're feeling light, happy and thinner. Take a nice walk today and know that you are reaping the benefits of keeping your skinny me in control. It's hard to believe that you let your fat self take over to begin with, especially when you know how much better you look and feel when you are your skinny self. The day is beautiful and so are you.

WHAT'S YOUR GOAL WEIGHT? _____
WHAT'S YOUR GOAL DATE? _____

Skinny me notebook lesson
I am beautiful because my skinny me is in control. 20 times.

Before starting day 15 refer back to your psych session and repeat the session again. You will do this at the beginning of every week.

DAY FIFTEEN (Monday)

Meditation for the day…Determination will be on the top of your skinny mind today. You are determined to shed that fat self forever. Look forward to the day when you can pass your fat clothes and this book onto another skinny friend trapped in their fat self. Today think about the advice you will give them as you hand over your past. Memorize and repeat this in your mind… "Determination for the duration is key for the skinny me."

WHAT'S YOUR GOAL WEIGHT? _____
WHAT'S YOUR GOAL DATE? _____

Skinny me notebook lesson
I am determined to shed the fat. 20 times.

DAY SIXTEEN (Tuesday)

Meditation for the day… In your mind picture a big fat trash can and visualize yourself throwing away all of the things associated with your fat self…first the layers and layers of fat, then the fear, depression, denial, anger, embarrassment, tears, self pity, jealousy, envy, pain, sickness and disease. Put a lid on it and let your skinny me dance away, feeling happy, light, healthy and beautiful.

WHAT'S YOUR GOAL WEIGHT? _____
WHAT'S YOUR GOAL DATE? _____

Skinny me notebook lesson
Tear out a page of your notebook and at the top put the heading "FAT SELF." Under the heading write down all of the things associated with the fat self as mentioned above. Wad it up and throw it away. Now, go back to your notebook and write: "I feel happy, light, healthy and beautiful." 20 times.

DAY SEVENTEEN (Wednesday)

Meditation for the day...Feel the power of positive thinking. You can do anything you put your mind to. Keep your skinny me in control and you will positively overpower your fat self. Positive people are in control and progress at a faster, healthier pace. Always find a positive within the negative and you'll overcome and feel good no matter what comes your way.

WHAT'S YOUR GOAL WEIGHT? _____
WHAT'S YOUR GOAL DATE? _____

Skinny me notebook lesson
Skinny me is positively in control. 20 times.

DAY EIGHTEEN (Thursday)

Meditation for the day... Think of your body as a working machine. You only need so much fuel to keep it working properly. Too much can cause the machine to flood out and eventually it can cause a total break down. The skinny me frame of mind knows its fuel intake limit and has an automatic shut off valve when it has had just enough. Never take in more fuel than you can burn or need to survive. Before you eat a meal, drink a glass of water. Eat slowly and concentrate on your stomach and how it feels after each and every bite. It may be satisfied after just a few bites. Stop eating and save the rest for later. Listen to your stomach and your skinny me.

WHAT'S YOUR GOAL WEIGHT? _____
WHAT'S YOUR GOAL DATE? _____

Skinny me notebook lesson
I know my fuel intake limit.   20 times.

DAY NINETEEN (Friday)

Meditation for the day… Every time you start to feel hungry today look at yourself in the mirror and into those eyes, remembering who is in control. Nobody else really cares if you side with your skinny self, in fact some people will try to discourage you and even try to trip you up just to make themselves feel better when you fail. Yes, sad but true this could even be your own family member. Stick with your skinny me, do it for yourself. You deserve it, you know you deserve it. Give yourself a big smile and a thank you for sticking with this program.

WHAT'S YOUR GOAL WEIGHT? _____
WHAT'S YOUR GOAL DATE? _____

Skinny me notebook lesson
I am sticking with my skinny me.　20 times.

DAY TWENTY (Saturday)

Meditation for the day... You've earned your own cheering section today. Pretend everyone is watching you and everything you put into your mouth. You hear the crowd cheering you on, backing you up and standing behind you 100%. You won't trip up because if you do you will see the disappointment on their faces. You'd rather cut off your big toe than to upset the crowd.

WHAT'S YOUR GOAL WEIGHT? _____
WHAT'S YOUR GOAL DATE? _____

Skinny me notebook lesson
I won't trip up. I am in control.   20 times.

DAY TWENTY-ONE (Sunday)

Meditation for the day… Your health test results are in and your doctor has just informed you that you suffer from a very curable illness called "Fat-ass-I-am." If you let it get out of control it can cause incurable diseases, such as diabetes, hypertension, heart disease, cancer and could eventually become fatal. All you have to do is follow the simple skinny me guidelines and your illness will go away completely.

WHAT'S YOUR GOAL WEIGHT? _____
WHAT'S YOUR GOAL DATE? _____

Skinny me notebook lesson
My skinny me will keep me healthy. 20 times.

DAY TWENTY-TWO (Monday)

Meditation for the day…Did you know you can dance while you are in a sitting position just by tightening your stomach and butt muscles to the beat of the music. In your car, in your bath, while you're laying in bed just before going to sleep…tune in and tone up, no matter where you are!

WHAT'S YOUR GOAL WEIGHT? _____
WHAT'S YOUR GOAL DATE? _____

Skinny me notebook lesson
I am motivated to move it and lose it.   20 times.

DAY TWENTY-THREE (Tuesday)

Meditation for the day… Visualize yourself lying comfortably in an oversized soft, cushioned hammock above snow-white sands in the shade beneath a grouping of massive palm trees on a deserted island. As you gaze out across the clear, light aqua blue ocean you hear the continuous soothing sounds of waves rolling onto shore. Amidst the light warm breeze you catch a faint scent of a familiar tropical suntan lotion and instantly you think to yourself, "damn, I wish I had a coconut cream pie." Not an option! I said this was a deserted island, not a dessert island. If you get a craving or start to reach for the wrong food, put yourself back into this hammock. If you fall off the hammock, refer to your "No need to sneak it" snack guide…be prepared, this could end up being your survival kit.

WHAT'S YOUR GOAL WEIGHT? _____
WHAT'S YOUR GOAL DATE? _____

Skinny me notebook lesson
My skinny me is in control of my destiny, therefore I am a survivor.   20 times.

DAY TWENTY-FOUR (Wednesday)

Meditation for the day… Have you seen yourself naked lately? Chances are you have, but what if every time you were in public and went to get a bite to eat your clothes would fall off? I think we would all make wiser choices of what we ate if we knew that everybody was going to see us in our birthday suits. Keep this in mind today when you reach for your food.

WHAT'S YOUR GOAL WEIGHT? _____
WHAT'S YOUR GOAL DATE? _____

Skinny me notebook lesson
My skinny me looks good with or without clothes. 20 times.

DAY TWENTY-FIVE (Thursday)

Meditation for the day... Have you seen your profile lately, head and all? Most people get a look at their front and back, but unless you have your mirrors adjusted just right, you don't really get the full impact of your profile. You may look like Alfred Hitchcock and not even be aware of it. Take some time today to get a good look at your profile. Compare it to other people you see today. Examine your neck area, stomach, butt, and thighs. When you are dancing today work up some new dance moves that target these specific areas. For the neck area it is as simple as tilting your head back and opening and closing your mouth wide enough to feel the stretch in your neck muscles. For your stomach, pull your muscles in and out. For your butt and thighs, tighten your muscles and squat up and down, just a slight motion will work wonders.

WHAT'S YOUR GOAL WEIGHT? _____
WHAT'S YOUR GOAL DATE? _____

Skinny me notebook lesson
I love what dancing does for my body, soul and mind.
20 times.

DAY TWENTY-SIX (Friday)

Meditation for the day…Your "skinny me" is watch dog for your innermost being. Skinny me will not let the negative in. So know today that positive prevails. Fatty can never touch your inner being without asking permission from your skinny me. Skinny me will not bend and will never give permission, because fatty is an inner being abuser. Stay focused on skinny me, your life depends on it.

WHAT'S YOUR GOAL WEIGHT? _____
WHAT'S YOUR GOAL DATE? _____

Skinny me notebook lesson
My skinny me stands guard 24/7.   20 times.

DAY TWENTY-SEVEN (Saturday)

Meditation for the day... Take time to laugh today. Your skinny me is telling fatty goodbye. Without looking back, without any regrets. You're visualizing the layers melting off. You're visualizing skinny me stepping out into the world, lean and laughing. Picture the lifestyle in which you are now placed as skinny me rather than fatty. Look who's laughing now. Start giving away that fat stuff, but don't forget to give your skinny friends who are still fighting to take control of fatty some advice on how to bring out their skinny me. This is a great feeling and we want everyone to feel as wonderful as we do.

WHAT'S YOUR GOAL WEIGHT? _____
WHAT'S YOUR GOAL DATE? _____

Skinny me notebook lesson
I'm laughing because I'm in control and I feel great. 20 times.

DAY TWENTY-EIGHT (Sunday)

Meditation for the day...Success is in the air around you. Skinny me has taken full control and you are reaping the benefits. Today when you reach for the sky take notice of God and thank him for keeping your skinny me strong. Reward yourself today, but don't let your guard down. Remember you are rewarding skinny me not fatty, so reward yourself with something that skinny me will appreciate.

WHAT'S YOUR GOAL WEIGHT? _____
WHAT'S YOUR GOAL DATE? _____

Skinny me notebook lesson
I thank God skinny me will always be in control. 20 times.

CHAPTER EIGHT

Everyday "SKINNY ME" Meals in Minutes

Use the products from your "SKINNY ME" PANTRY & FRIDGE LIST: Be sure to use your "Don't be a pig about it" portion control chart when preparing and consuming your meals.

GUILT FREE DRINKS FOR ANY MEAL:

green tea (hot or iced), mineral water (may be flavored with natural fruit juice), tap or spring water, coffee (black or with skim milk).

Don't forget how important it is to have those six to eight glasses of water per day. Try to stay away from diet soda, which contains fake sugars. If you can't resist, try to at least restrain. Ask your "skinny self" first if she/he would prefer water over diet soda...the answer will be:

"Yes, you inconsiderate cow!"

BREAKFAST ideas:

SIMPLICITY breakfast
1 grapefruit or 1 cup of berries
1 slice whole grain toast, bagel, or English muffin with
1 pat butter or 2 teaspoons cream cheese, 1 serving of
hot or cold cereal of your choice

MIX IT UP breakfast
2 slices whole grain toast or 1 English muffin or 1
bagel with 2 tablespoons cream cheese topped with
fresh strawberry slices

WAKE ME UP breakfast
In a skillet, heat on medium high heat:
1 tablespoon of olive oil
Toss in ½ cup broccoli florets

In a bowl, scramble a couple of egg whites with two
tablespoons skim milk, one tablespoon diced red or green
bell peppers and a dash of salt, a dash or two of cayenne
pepper, and ½ teaspoon chili powder. Pour mixture over
the broccoli and scramble together. While it is still cooking,
squeeze some fresh lime juice on it. When it is cooked, add
3 tablespoons of your favorite shredded cheese. Wrap it
up in a whole grain tortilla or serve it straight up on a plate.
If you are really hungry, you can add 2 ounces of meat or
one slice of bacon. If you can't handle spicy foods, omit
the cayenne pepper and use black pepper in its place.

LET's GO breakfast

1 serving of hot or cold cereals (choose one full of fiber and use skim milk when you prepare it)

One cup of your favorite fruit

One slice of whole grain toast

TREAT ME breakfast (limit this item to once a week)

Three 4" pancakes with berries cooked in or on the side (use a light or gluten free pancake mix, the kind you mix with water or skim milk)

Use real maple syrup and limit yourself to 3 tablespoons and one pat of butter

SWEET, SMOOTH & NUTRITIONAL breakfast

Mix in a blender:

1 cup orange juice or pineapple juice

3/4 cup frozen berry mix (blackberries, strawberries, raspberries)

1/2 banana

If you need a solid food with this, have a 1/2 whole grain bagel with a tablespoon of cream cheese.

Café breakfast:

Bottled water and an egg on an English muffin or wheat toast. Fruit dish and or yogurt

LUNCH ideas:

Lite & Filling Lunch
4 tablespoons of chicken salad or tuna salad on a whole
grain tortilla or low carb whole grain bread...toast and
add some lettuce. Mix in a few chopped almonds for
texture.
One cup of raw veggies
One apple, peach or plum
One 8 oz. cup of skim milk or iced raspberry green tea

Simple Salad Lunch
1 small broiled, baked or grilled chicken breast chopped
into small cubes or strips
2-3 cups lettuce (spring mix or romaine works best)
1 tablespoon dried cranberries or 4 fresh strawberries
sliced
5 pecan halves
brocccoli sprouts (to your desired taste)
1 tablespoon olive oil mixed with 1 tablespoon balsamic
vinegar and 1/4 teaspoon honey

Back at School Lunch
2 slices of whole grain bread toasted and spread with:
2 tablespoons whole peanut butter (no sugar added)
1 tablespoon 100% fruit spread or 3-4 slices of fresh
strawberries or 4-6 grapes, halved

Hot Veggie Lunch
In a large microwave-safe bowl with lid, mix together

1-3 small chopped red potatoes, some broccoli, carrots, and fresh green beans or pea pods, 1/4 teaspoon basil, crushed garlic and one teaspoon olive oil and sprinkle a little parmesan cheese on top. Pour in 3 tablespoons of water, place the lid on and microwave for about two to two-and-a-half minutes until veggies are done. (This is great to take to the office already prepared and microwave there at lunchtime…you can also eat as much as you want, but no more than three small potatoes.)

DINNER tips:

Use your "Skinny" sense and eat a healthy meal, however if you are craving junk food or fast food have another go at the drive through lunch routine I mentioned earlier. A few days of this will break you of that bad habit. Also, stick with the basics: 1 portion of protein, 1-3 portions of steamed vegies, 1 portion of fruit and 1 slice of whole grain bread. Listen to your stomach, when it tells you it is "full" don't keep stuffing your pie hole.

"NO NEED TO SNEAK IT" SNACK GUIDE

Baked Garlic
1 or 2 full heads of garlic, trim off all points and peel off outer skin, leaving just enough skin to hold the garlic together.

Place the garlic in a small baking dish along with 3 tablespoons of white wine or orange juice, and one-and-a-half teaspoons olive oil.

Bake at 350 degrees for one hour. You can bake this ahead of time and keep it in the fridge until you want to eat it, just take off a few cloves and microwave for a few seconds until it is warm again, or eat it cold.

TIP: Use this in place of butter and eat it on whole grain Melba toast, coupled with goat cheese or cream cheese. I like to put this out as an appetizer along with some fresh sprigs of Thyme.

Nutty & Fruity
2 tablespoons all natural peanut butter with NO ADDED SUGAR, spread onto apple slices, celery sticks or whole grain Melba toast with fresh strawberry slices

Berry Wrap
One half whole grain tortilla
2 tablespoons of cream cheese

4 strawberries sliced
Heat the tortilla for 14 seconds in the microwave, spread on cream cheese and strawberries then roll it up and enjoy.

Pear Pleaser
1 pear sliced into thin strips
1 serving size hard Parmesan cheese or asiago cheese sliced into thin wafers
Place the cheese onto the pear slices.

Salsa Tortilla
2 plum tomatoes, chopped
1 small yellow or white onion
1/2 teaspoon oregano
1 tablespoon lime juice
1 tablespoon cilantro
You may spice this up with some jalapeno pepper slices
You can also mix up a larger batch of this salsa and keep in the fridge up to 1 week.

Warm up a whole grain tortilla and spread it with cream cheese or strips of cooked, sliced chicken breast. Top with salsa and roll up.

You don't have to be an Egyptian to live by the food pyramid. Look at it daily as a reminder of how you should eat.

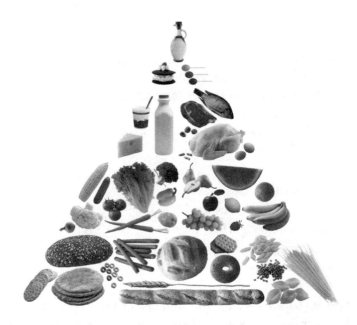

DAILY:

Fats & Oils: try olive oil or canola (sparingly)

Sweets: naturally sweet, light or low fat (sparingly)

Milk, Yogurt & Cheese: skim or low fat (2-3 servings)

Fruits: fresh is best (2-4 servings)

Veggies: fresh or steamed (3-5 servings)

Bread, Cereal, Rice & Pasta: whole grain or sprouted grain (6-11 servings) cut back on this group for a better weight loss.

COUNT those CALORIES!!!

CHAPTER NINE

"Don't be a Pig about it"

Keep from being a pig with the help of these size relations on portions...

1 portion =

- Fats: your thumb tip

- Cheese: a pair of dice

- Skim Milk or Yogurt: one fist

- Ice Cream: 1/2 baseball

- Meat, Fish or Poultry: deck of cards

- Vegetables or Fruit: a baseball

- Steamed rice: 1/2 baseball

- Pasta: 1/2 baseball

- Potato: 1/2 baseball

- Bagel: a hockey puck

- Pancake: a compact disc

- Snack foods: 1/2 baseball

"Skinny me" Serving Sizes:

- 1 slice of whole-grain bread *(anymore and you're a PIG!)*

- 1/2 cup of cooked rice or pasta *(anymore and you're a PIG!)*

- 1/2 cup of mashed potatoes *(anymore and you're a PIG!)*

- 3-4 small crackers *(anymore and you're a PIG!)*

- 1 small pancake or waffle *(anymore and you're a PIG!)*

- 2 medium-sized cookies *(anymore and you're a PIG!)*

- 1/2 cup cooked vegetables *(anymore and you're a PIG!)*

- 1 cup (4 leaves) lettuce *(anymore and you're a PIG!)*

- 1 small baked potato *(anymore and you're a PIG!)*

- 3/4 cup vegetable juice *(anymore and you're a PIG!)*

- 1 medium apple *(anymore and you're a PIG!)*

- 1/2 grapefruit or mango *(anymore and you're a PIG!)*

- 1/2 cup berries *(anymore and you're a PIG!)*

- 1 cup yogurt or milk *(anymore and you're a PIG!)*

- 1 1/2 ounces of cheddar cheese *(anymore and you're a PIG!)*

- 1 chicken breast *(anymore and you're a PIG!)*

- 1 medium pork chop *(anymore and you're a PIG!)*

- 1/4 pound hamburger patty *(anymore and you're a PIG!)*

CHAPTER TEN

You Make the Choice

VERY IMPORTANT!!! You should keep this book on hand at all times. Everyday, before you eat anything, open this book to this chapter and review the following photos. You have a choice, and these photos should keep your Skinny Self in check. This is your "Skinny Me" opportunity to take control. Do it now! Each day, before you leave your home, stuff this book into your purse or car before "Fatty" stuffs it in a drawer.

Do you want to be your **FAT** Self?
    or
Do you want to be your **SKINNY** Self?

Your Choose...

Listen to your **FAT SELF** and look like this

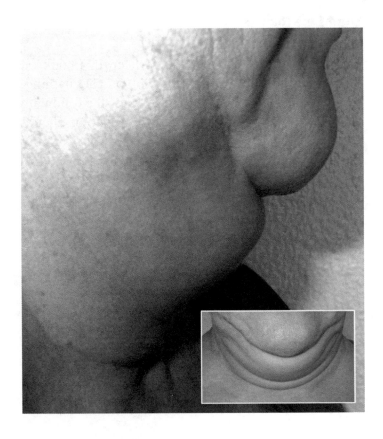

What the hell is that thing?

Do you suffer from Neckrolliosis? *(also known as "foreskin of the face" or "Hangjollijaw")*

Listen to your **SKINNY SELF** and look like this ▼

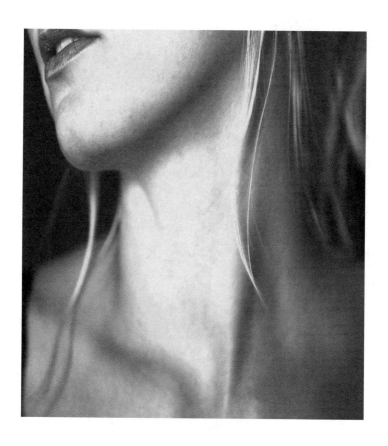

The Choice is Yours.

Listen to your **FAT SELF** and look like this

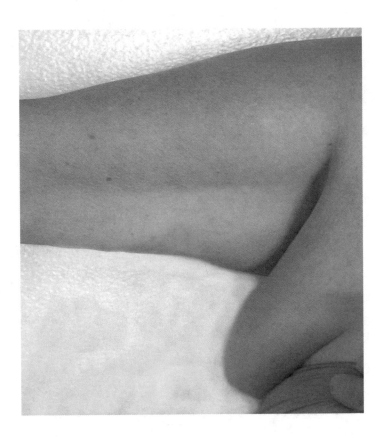

It must have been "add-a-titt-by-my-pit" day at the ballpark. Were you there?

Listen to your **SKINNY SELF** and look like this ▼

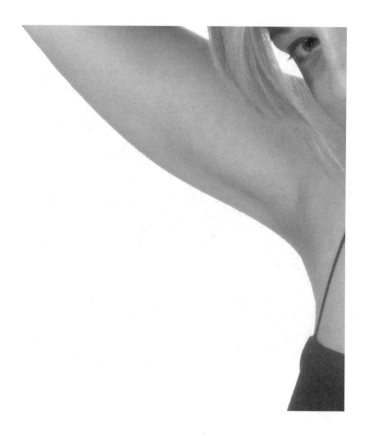

The Choice is Yours.

Listen to your **FAT SELF** and look like this

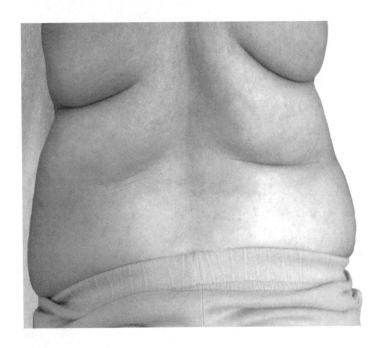

Do you want your loved ones to accidentally cop a feel of this when they greet you hello or goodbye? Gross.

Listen to your **SKINNY SELF** and look like this ▼

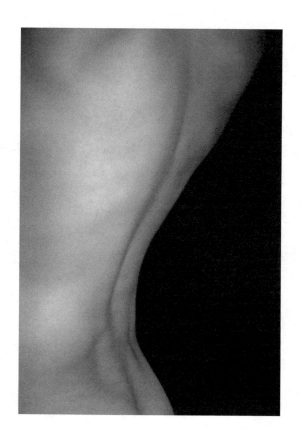

The Choice is Yours.

Listen to your **FAT SELF** and look like this

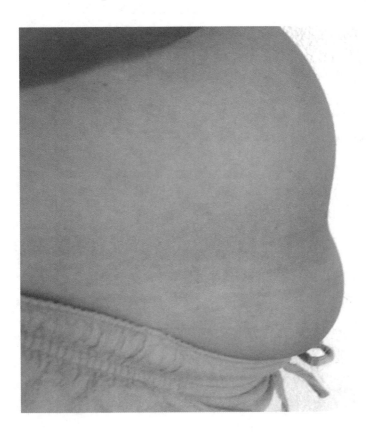

The "I'm just bloated" excuse will not work if you look like this.

"I'm pregnant" might work, or "I have a melon lodged between my upper and lower intestines.

80

Listen to your **SKINNY SELF** and look like this

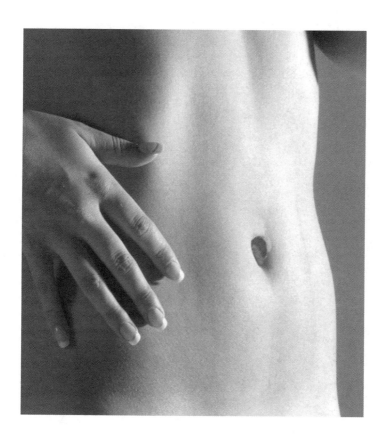

The Choice is Yours.

Listen to your **FAT SELF** and look like this

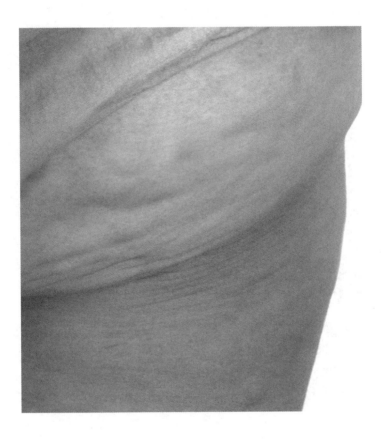

Have you ever looked at the surface of the moon through a high powered telescope?

Cottage cheese anyone?

Listen to your **SKINNY SELF** and look like this

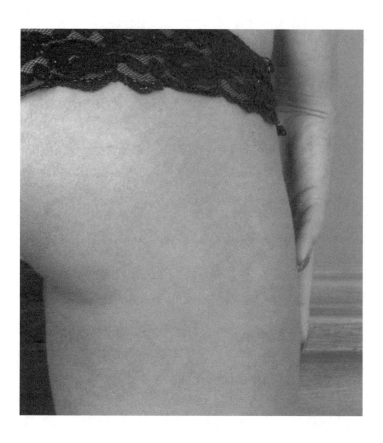

The Choice is Yours.

Listen to your **FAT SELF** and look like this

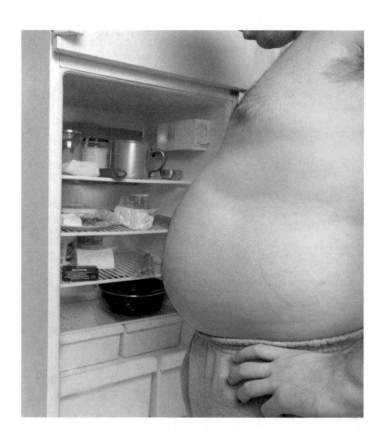

To hell with the baked chicken, I'm going for the beer, brats, beans, buns, apple pie and then another beer.

Listen to your **SKINNY SELF** and look like this

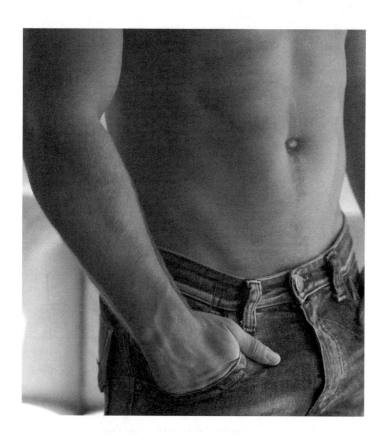

The Choice is Yours.

"Skinny Me" lesson

"Skinny Me" lesson

"Skinny Me" lesson

"Skinny Me" lesson

"Skinny Me" lesson

"Skinny Me" lesson

"Skinny Me" lesson

"Skinny Me" lesson

"Skinny Me" lesson

"Skinny Me" lesson

"Skinny Me" lesson

"Skinny Me" lesson

"Skinny Me" lesson

"Skinny Me" lesson

"Skinny Me" lesson

"Skinny Me" lesson

"Skinny Me" lesson

"Skinny Me" lesson

"Skinny Me" lesson

"Skinny Me" lesson

"Skinny Me" lesson

"Skinny Me" lesson

"Skinny Me" lesson

"Skinny Me" lesson

"Skinny Me" lesson

"Skinny Me" lesson

"Skinny Me" lesson

"Skinny Me" lesson